PRACTICAL GUIDE 2 ADDICTION THERAPY

Developed for therapists, counselors, recovering addicts, and parents or significant others of recovering addicts

DR JOSEPH ADEGBOYEGA

TABLE OF CONTENTS

SERENITY PRAYER

God grant me the Serenity to accept the things I cannot change,
Courage to change the things I can,
And the Wisdom to know the difference.

Living one day at a time,
Enjoying one moment at a time,
Accepting hardship as the pathway to peace.

Taking, as He did, this Sinful World as it is,
not as I would have it;

Trusting that He will make all things right if I surrender to
His will;

That I may be reasonably happy in this life, And supremely
happy with Him forever in the next.

BY REINHOLD NIEBUHR – 1892 - 1971

Researched and prepared by:

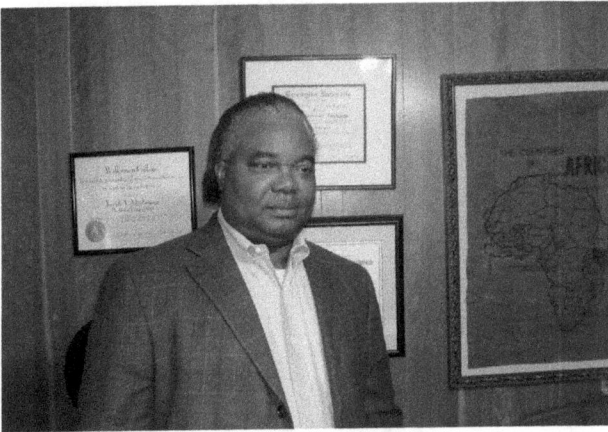

Joseph Adegboyega (Dr. Joe), PhD, MAC, LCAS, CCS, SAP

Dr. Joe is a licensed clinical addiction specialist, internationally certified advanced alcohol and drug counselor, certified clinical supervisor, and substance abuse professional (USDOT).

Note: _Patients' names used herein are fictitious, but the stories are true._

APPRECIATION/GRATITUDE:

Praises to the Creator for the various blessings, gratitude to my father (Raphael Adegboyega) for the love, to my mother (Mrs. Esther Biola Adegboyega) for the love, to my wife and friend (Mrs. Veronica Halter-Adegboyega, a.k.a. "Mama Ve") for the love and support, to Mr. Felix Akinjo (headmaster at St. Matthew's Primary School, Ondo Nigeria) for the discipline and lessons of life, to my many primary school teachers (Papa Adegoke, Pa Akindoju, etc.) for the education, to my local and foreign teachers (Reverend Brothers of the De La Salle Order, Canada) at St. Joseph Secondary School, Ondo, for a quality high school education, to my various teachers at the University of Nice and University of Toulouse France (special thanks to Professor Pierre Velas) for the excellent university education, and to Monsieur Marcel Entressangle of Nice, France, for giving me a job at a crucial time following my arrival in Nice. I thank my ex-wife (Josiane née Rateau) for her support during those years in France and in Nigeria. I thank every man and woman who along the way gave me support, however small.

TOPIC 1.

WHAT IS DRUG ADDICTION TREATMENT?

There are many addictive drugs and mood-altering substances. Treatment for specific drugs/substances can differ. Treatment also varies depending on the characteristics of the patient.

Therapists should endeavor to meet the recovering drug addict wherever he or she might be, for several reasons:

- Problems associated with an individual's drug addiction can vary significantly,

- Recovering drug addicts come from different walks of life, and

- Consideration must be given to family history of mental illness, occupation, health, and the severity of the addiction, plus social problems make treatment much more difficult to treat.

BEHAVIORAL THERAPY: Drug addiction treatment includes behavioral therapy (such as counseling, cognitive therapy, or psychotherapy), medications, or a combination of the two. Behavioral therapies teach drug addicts strategies for avoiding drugs and preventing relapse and can help them deal with relapse when it occurs. Drug addicts are at a higher risk for AIDS and other infectious diseases; in this case, behavioral therapies can help reduce the risk of disease transmission and infection. Case management and referrals to services such as medical, psychological, and social services take into consideration a holistic approach (the needs of the patient as a whole) to drug addiction treatment. Studies show that the best programs provide a combination of therapies and other services to address the needs of the individual patient. Treatment for addiction can include medications, behavioral therapy, or a combination of the two.

Meeting the patient wherever he or she might be takes into consideration issues such as age, race, culture, sexual orientation, gender, pregnancy, parenting, housing, and employment, as well as physical and sexual abuse.

MEDICATIONS: Treatment with medications, such as methadone, LAAM, and naltrexone, are available for individuals addicted to opiates. Nicotine preparations (patches, gum, or nasal spray) and bupropion are available for individuals addicted to nicotine (tobacco products).

Components of Comprehensive Drug Abuse Treatment

The best treatment programs provide a combination of therapies and other services to meet the needs of the individual patient.

Individual patient needs could be all or some of the following: child care services, vocational services, mental health services, medical services, educational services, AIDS/HIV services, legal services, financial services, housing/transportation services, and family services.

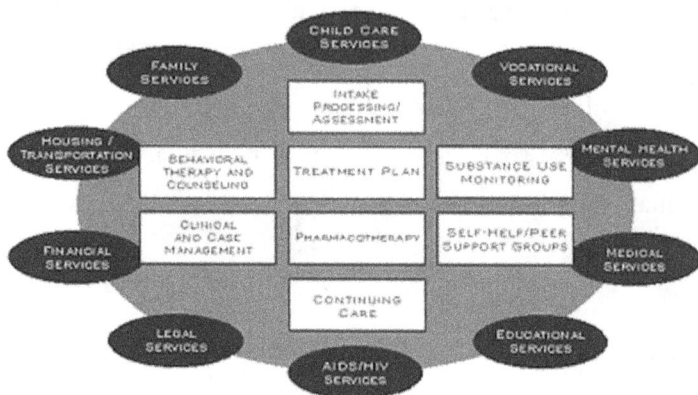

(Courtesy of DrugAbuse.gov)

For dually diagnosed patients, such as individuals suffering from co-occurring mental disorders such as depression, anxiety disorder, bipolar disorder, or psychosis, medications such as antidepressants, mood stabilizers, or neuroleptics may be critical for treatment success. Treatment can occur in a variety of settings, in many different forms, and for different lengths of time. Because drug addiction is typically a chronic disorder characterized by occasional relapses, a short-term, one-time treatment often is not sufficient. For many, treatment is a long-term process that involves multiple interventions and attempts at abstinence.

<u>Note:</u> *Therapists should caution the recovering addict to endeavor to attend therapy sessions and not rely on medications alone.*

WHY CAN'T DRUG ADDICTS QUIT ON THEIR OWN?

DENIAL AND FALLACY: Most drug addicts believe falsely that they *can* quit on their own, thereby minimizing the severity of the addiction. Many addicted individuals believe in the beginning that they can stop using drugs on their own, and most try to stop without treatment but in vain. Unfortunately, most attempts to quit result in failure to achieve abstinence for a long period of time. Chronic drug addiction often results in deep and permanent damage to the brain. Once brain functions are severely altered, the individual is then prone to use drugs despite adverse consequences (the compulsion to use), which is the defining characteristic of addiction. Try this experiment: take two balloons and inflate one. Continue to inflate the balloon over and over. Take note that the balloon that was not inflated maintains the same steady and uniform structure, whereas the balloon that was inflated repeatedly presents a wrinkled structure. This is what happens to a brain that has been subjected to several substance-induced highs.

Studies show that stress from work and family and other environmental factors and events are likely triggers for relapse. However, there is hope that with active participation in treatment, an individual is likely to succeed in attaining long-term abstinence.

<u>Note:</u> *Denial is huge in the early stage of recovery. The therapist must work with the recovering addict in order to help him or her overcome denial.*

TRUE STORY: Debbie, a thirty-nine-year-old white banker, successfully completed a methadone medication-assisted therapy program at a methadone clinic. Debbie took methadone from low to high doses and was eventually weaned off of the drug by the time she graduated. Debbie remained abstinent for many months and was eventually able to live life to the fullest, without the use of mood-altering substances.

TOPIC 2.

WHAT ROLE CAN THE CRIMINAL JUSTICE SYSTEM PLAY?

Integration of the criminal justice system with community-based treatment is increasingly showing positive results in helping drug addicts turn their lives around. Studies show that treatment for drug-addicted offenders during and after incarceration can have a significant beneficial effect upon future drug use, criminal behavior, and social functioning. *(For example, a recent study found that prisoners who participated in a therapeutic treatment program in the Delaware State Prison and continued to receive treatment in a work-release program after prison were 70 percent less likely than nonparticipants to return to drug use and incur rearrest.)*

Studies show that drug addicts who enter treatment via the criminal justice system achieve comparable levels of success to those who enter treatment voluntarily.

The criminal justice system refers drug offenders into treatment through a variety of mechanisms, such as diverting nonviolent offenders to treatment, stipulating treatment as a condition of probation or pretrial release, and convening specialized courts that handle cases for offenses involving drugs. Drug courts, another model, are dedicated to drug offender cases. They mandate and arrange for treatment as an alternative to incarceration, actively monitoring progress in treatment and arranging for other services to drug-involved offenders.

The most effective models integrate criminal justice and drug treatment systems and services. Treatment and criminal justice personnel work together on plans and implementation of screening, placement, testing, monitoring, and supervision, as well as on the systematic use of sanctions and rewards for drug abusers in the criminal justice system. Treatment for incarcerated drug abusers must include continuing care, monitoring, and supervision after release and during parole.

Note: _The therapist might suggest a visit to drug court or the local detention center to encourage the recovering addict to appreciate the need for him or her to commit to treatment._

TRUE STORY: Jason, a thirty-one-year-old unemployed black male, was a drug dealer and drug user. He was arrested for possession with intent to distribute. Until he was facing drug charges, it was difficult for Jason to admit that he was addicted to both the money and the drugs. Once Jason realized that he could be sent to prison for some time, he quickly took a plea bargain for probation and treatment.

TRIGGERS: PEOPLE, PLACES, AND EVENTS

The human brain associates particular feelings with people, places, and events. This intertwined mental association often causes drug addicts to relapse. At any stage during recovery, particularly in the early stages, the drug addict could be triggered to use due to old feelings, people, places, and events. Unless the drug addict takes action to prevent cravings and possible relapse, he or she is extremely vulnerable to returning to using or drinking. The addict must avoid known external and obvious triggers. The addict in recovery has to anticipate and prepare to neutralize any triggers that arise.

PEOPLE: Draw a list of people who could serve as a trigger for relapse (for example, your relatives, your spouse, your girlfriend or boyfriend, your children, your boss, your coworkers, your neighbors, and any others).

PLACES: What places could trigger cravings or euphoric recall? Make a list of the places that might remind you of drinking/using (for example, bars, clubs, golf courses, football games and tailgating, school, work, certain streets, concerts, pool halls, certain country roads, lakes, backyards, and so on).

EVENTS: What routine events could trigger cravings? Make a list of possible trigger-provoking events (for example, fishing, mowing the lawn, fundraising events, gambling, attending music festivals, and others).

CELEBRATIONS: Celebrations or special events can trigger relapse (such as weddings, graduations, birthdays, vacations, and holidays).

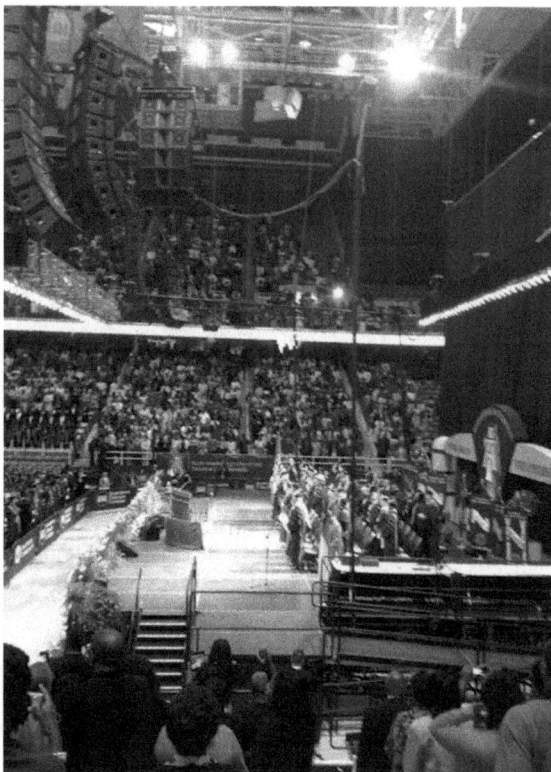

Graduation ceremony at NC A&T
University, Greensboro, NC, 2012

OTHER STRESSFUL EVENTS OR ACTIVITIES:
List other stressful events or activities that could trigger
relapse, such as deaths of family members, divorce, separation, money problems, getting paid, getting a raise, calls
from creditors, paying bills, group meetings, long work

hours, unemployment, having a baby, retiring, being home alone, being on vacation, going by an ATM machine, finding paraphernalia, and so on.

RELATIONSHIP EVENTS: Relationship events can serve as a trigger (for example, meeting new people, going out on a date, hanging out with friends, arguments, sex, viewing pornography, family visits, having a baby, separation, and so on).

TIME: Certain times of the day, week, month, or year might trigger relapse, such as, Monday night football or Sundays (gearing up to go back to work).

Note: The therapist must encourage the recovering addict to plan to be assertive and empower him or herself to escape whenever he or she feels trapped.

TRUE STORY: Michael, a twenty-seven-year-old single white male, was the son of a popular attorney in California. Michael had struggled with drug addiction for years. He had received treatment at more than two residential treatment centers using a combination of medication and therapy. After the last treatment, Michael was abstinent from drugs for over two years. Michael was planning to resume his college education when he attended a party with his girlfriend. While at the party, Michael made the fatal mistake of accepting an alcoholic drink and later did some drugs before slipping into a coma. Michael was rushed to the hospital, and he later died. Michael's parents and sibling were devastated.

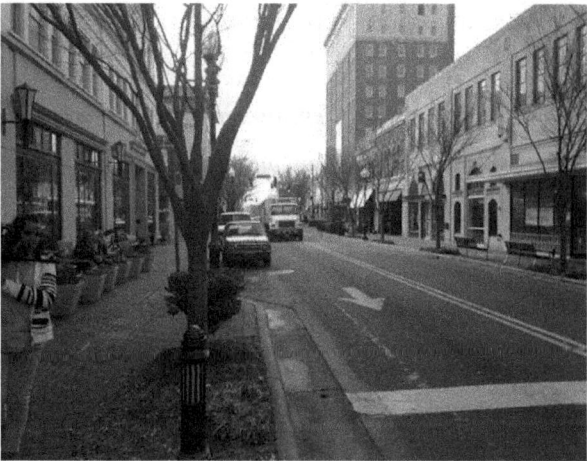

Substances of Abuse : Pictures of downtown Winston Salem, NC, showing bars and restaurants

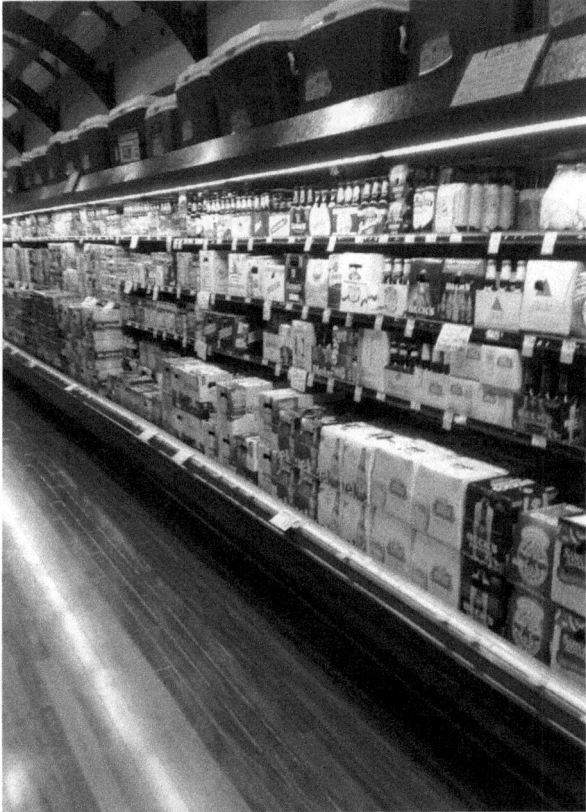

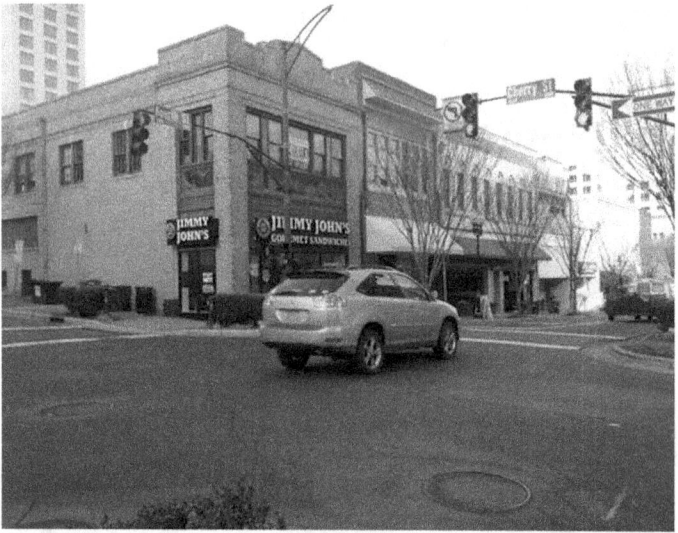

Pictures of downtown Winston Salem, NC,
showing bars and restaurants

TOPIC 4.

DRUG URGES (CRAVINGS)

There are varying shapes and forms to addictions and cravings, but they all stem from a fancy piece of the mesolimbic system in the brain. The mesolimbic system is the brain's reward or reinforcement center. It says "nice job!" when you do something good or pleasurable by releasing dopamine, a chemical that makes you feel good.

Dopamine is a group of twenty-two atoms: eight carbon, eleven hydrogen, one nitrogen, and two oxygen ($C_8H_{11}NO_2$).

"The pleasure associated and the rewards from certain behaviors...all seem to involve dopamine," says Dr. Andrew Moorhouse at The University of New South Wales.

When we do something pleasurable, such as eating or having sex, the brain processes positive stimuli, and dopamine is released very deep in our brain, in the nucleus accumbens. When the brain rewards certain behaviors, the impulse to repeat such behaviors becomes the reinforcement that the behavior is good. This is how the compulsion to use drugs grows!

<u>Note:</u> *Honesty in treatment is very important. The therapist has to encourage the recovering addict to be honest about cravings and the urges to use.*

TRUE STORY: Jeff, a forty-two-year-old black male painter was receiving drug treatment and had been abstinent. After a lull of three months, Jeff started to report periodic cravings for drugs. Jeff was able to surmount these cravings a couple of times. What helped Jeff was that he discussed his concerns with his therapist. The therapist prepared some relapse-prevention strategies with Jeff. Jeff finally agreed to a safety plan with the therapist: he would call a supportive person or a sponsor, engage in outdoor activities until the cravings passed, meditate or do yoga, write in his journal, or find people/friends to talk to when the cravings hit.

TOPIC 5.

INFECTIOUS DISEASE RISK REDUCTION

Drug addicts, such as heroin or cocaine addicts, and particularly injection (IV) drug users, are at an increased risk for HIV/AIDS as well as other infectious diseases like hepatitis, tuberculosis, and sexually transmitted infections. Drug addiction treatment targeting these individuals is vital for community disease prevention. In other words, drug abuse treatment is also disease prevention.

Studies show that IV drug users who do not enter treatment are up to six times more likely to become infected with HIV than injectors who enter and remain in treatment. Active participation in drug treatment helps to reduce the spread of diseases. It is well known that sharing injection equipment and engaging in unprotected sexual activities contribute to the spread of diseases. Treatment also presents opportunities for screening, counseling, and referrals for additional services. HIV counseling and HIV testing are criteria of the best drug abuse treatment programs.

Note: The therapist must encourage the recovering addict to get tested for infectious diseases. Knowing whether or not he or she is infected will help curb the spread of diseases.

TRUE STORY: Alcohol and drugs loosen inhibitions, making people more open to risky sexual activities. Becky, a twenty-six-year-old single black female, went out with her girlfriend to watch sporting events with some male acquaintances. Everyone present was consuming alcohol as they watched the games. Later that night, Becky's girlfriend sensed danger, and she decided to leave. Becky, who was also drinking, decided to stay. Shortly after Becky's friend left the scene, Becky agreed to have sex with a new guy she met at the party. As Becky and the man were having sex, they were surprised by three other men who rushed into the room to join in. Becky was repeatedly raped by three—or more—men from the party. Becky passed out in shock and was rushed to the hospital.

TOPIC 6.

FAMILY INVOLVEMENT

The involvement of family members and the need to fellowship with loving or supportive people are prerequisites for success in drug treatment. In many successful and effective drug treatment programs, family and friends play critical roles in motivating individuals to enter and stay in treatment. Family therapy is important, especially for adolescents. The involvement of a family member in an individual's treatment program can strengthen and extend the benefits of the program. The patient who readily accepts family involvement in treatment tends to be more accountable.

Note: _The therapist must encourage the recovering drug addict to involve family members in the treatment. The involvement of supportive loved ones is likely to provide better monitoring of changes in behavior, preempt relapse, and enhance progress._

TRUE STORY: Karen, a forty-five-year-old white single mother, entered into drug treatment. Karen was receiving financial support from her parents, who took her in following her divorce from her husband. It was necessary for Karen to demonstrate to her parents that she was compliant, plus the parents were well positioned to provide corroborating information on Karen's recovery efforts. It was therefore necessary for Karen to involve her parents for proper monitoring of her behavior during treatment. Family involvement is crucial for success in outpatient treatment settings. In many cases when the patient declines to involve parents or family, it is often because the patient wants to be in control and not be accountable to anyone.

TOPIC 7.

RELATIONSHIPS IN RECOVERY

Falling in love can have a negative effect on recovery. Sex can awaken the "sleeping giant" in the addict. The "sleeping giant" is the backlog of unmet emotional needs from previous relationships. Unmet emotional needs reside in the unconscious and are sealed off from our awareness. At the least, one year of sobriety and relationship abstinence is necessary to allow the recovering addict to deal with his or her own emotions, build on self-awareness, and take control of his or her own emotions. The recovering addict begins to rely on his or herself as a source of emotional nourishment and strength, rather than relying on an external source for relief or emotional gain, which is what he or she is accustomed to doing.

"The most important relationship is with oneself": this concept poses a complete paradigm shift to the recovering drug addict. If the necessary amount of time to grow the relationship with oneself hasn't lapsed, chances are that the recovering addict will do whatever he or she is accustomed to doing during crisis. The recovering drug addict will look outside of his or herself for relief or to make up for what is "missing" emotionally.

Note: *The therapist must remind the recovering drug addict to steer clear of forming relationships during recovery, particularly in the early stages of recovery.*

TRUE STORY: Sarah, a twenty-seven-year-old black college student, is a perfect cautionary tale for not getting into relationships in early recovery. One of Sarah's experiences turned out very ugly. Five years ago Sarah decided to move in with a man she'd recently met, John. They both had been sober for only a few months. About one month later, Sarah was in the ER, drunk and pretty roughed up. Sarah was very lucky. John had almost killed the last two female friends he had been with. Sarah didn't know that John had served time in detention. Sarah was scared to death, but she pressed charges, and John ended up back in jail. Sarah received a lot of counseling at the ER that night. She was offered resources for recovery from alcoholism. Sarah was very lucky to be alive to tell this story in treatment; too many relationships end fatally.

TOPIC 8.

SOCIAL LIFE AND SOCIAL PRESSURE TO USE

The addict in recovery must learn to say "no" in social situations. Social pressures to use drugs can be very strong, and the recovering addict has to be strong and assertive enough to say "no" when pressured to use or drink. Young people are particularly vulnerable to pressures from peers. Some children are susceptible to influence from their parents to use alcohol, tobacco, and other drugs. The strong "pull" or desire to belong might push young people to succumb to pressures to use drugs. It must be noted that a different set of pressures exist for those involved in competitive sports or bodybuilding. They may use substances, particularly anabolic steroids, because they view such drug use as an accepted part of a successful training regimen.

Note: Social pressures to use drugs or alcohol are difficult to fight. The therapist must encourage the recovering drug addict to avoid certain social circles during and after treatment.

TRUE STORY: Sam, a thirty-nine-year-old white rock musician and single father, was a recovering chronic heroin addict. Sam was receiving treatment in an outpatient setting and had been abstinent, using Suboxone for about nine months. Deep into his recovery, Sam joined a new band. The band played to a big crowd one night, and after the show the band members decided to celebrate. Sam found himself sitting in a circle with fellow band members. The band members started to pass drugs around, and each member hit the "cigar" a couple of times. Sam did as well and regretted it. But it was too late. Sam stated that he was high for several hours. Sam was devastated as he contemplated the ramifications of his relapse. Since he had entered into treatment, Sam had regained sole custody of his only child. Sam's therapist processed the "slip" with him so as to prepare him to survive the next temptation.

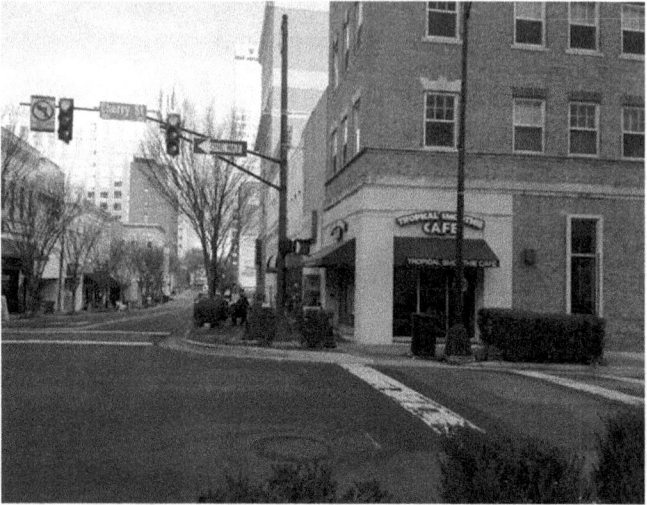

Picture of downtown Winston Salem, NC,
showing bars and restaurants

USE OF OTHER DRUGS

Some addicts in recovery might indulge in abstinence by substitution. This is defined as substituting one substance or habit for another (for example, substituting a cocaine addiction for sex, shopping, or gambling). It is best to help the recovering addict find activities to cope with boredom or fill the void within.

Note: The urge to switch from one substance to another is particularly great at the initial stage. The therapist should instruct and prepare the recovering drug addict to work hard at total abstinence and not substitute one substance for another.

TRUE STORY: While working at a methadone clinic, a therapist and his team observed that many patients who had entered into treatment for chronic opioid dependence started testing positive for cocaine. The use of other drugs started once the recovering addicts had attained several weeks of abstinence from the opioid. Studies show that most people with addictive personalities will often switch from one substance to another or from one behavior to another. It is therefore possible that an addict will switch from gambling to shopping, or from cocaine to heroin, or from marijuana to cocaine.

IDENTIFYING THE RELAPSE PROCESS

The best treatment approach is to assist the recovering addict in identifying the relapse process and to equip him or her with strategies to deal appropriately with future incidents.

Note: Relapse is an integral part of recovery. It is important that the therapist, soon after a relapse episode, helps the recovering drug addict to identify the relapse process in order to prepare him or her for future incidents.

TRUE STORY: Sandra, a thirty-three-year-old black banker, relapsed for some days. Recognizing that relapse is part of recovery, Sandra did not waste time in contacting her therapist for assistance. With the help of her therapist, Sandra walked back in her mind, trying to understand how and why she relapsed.

TOPIC 11.

PARTICIPATION IN THE TWELVE-STEP PROGRAM

The recovering drug addict should be encouraged to attend support group meetings. Such meetings provide opportunities to share and learn from others in recovery. There are several groups for recovering addicts and their loved ones, such as AA (Alcoholics Anonymous), NA (Narcotics Anonymous), and CA (Cocaine Anonymous)). In general, most programs are based on AA's twelve-step model of recovery. Participation during and after treatment should be encouraged.

Note: Participation in support group meetings is crucial for long-term abstinence and recovery. Without prompting and encouragement, very few recovering addicts would choose to attend NA or AA meetings. It is therefore important that the therapist, in the early stages of recovery, discuss with the recovering addict the benefits of participating in support group meetings.

TRUE STORY: Bryan, a forty-two-year-old black businessman, completed outpatient treatment without problems and remained abstinent for six months after discharge. As Bryan was being discharged, he was instructed to endeavor to attend support group meetings. Bryan failed to attend any until he relapsed due to pressure from his business. The therapist again encouraged Bryan to start attending support group meetings, to start to learn from other addicts, and to share his experience in recovery with others.

SPIRITUALITY IN RECOVERY

Faith and spirituality are important factors in recovery. Recovery is often sustained by spirituality.

What is spirituality? It is the spirit in me. It's in you...and in all of us in all realms of existence. Religion is a set of behaviors, or actions we take, relevant to our belief system and/or faith. Religion is designed to help the state of humankind improve spiritually. Whereas religion can be limiting, *spirit* is what we are. Thus spirit is unlimited. Spirituality is the practice of being who we are: the connection of all into a "oneness." Spiritual practice is defined as a set of things we do to help us connect with who we are and bring clarity to reality. Reality is defined as what is behind everything that we see, touch, smell, and hear.

Humans give different names to reality, such God, Buddha, Allah, Divine Mother, Great Spirit, Krishna, or the Tao.

Nobody knows the true nature of reality. The evidence of reality is sometimes seen in the transformation of people and things—when they have been touched by God (reality) in such a way that nothing else could.

God the Creator reveals him or herself to each of us in many different ways. Each one of us understands God independently, separately, and individually.

Note: Faith and spirituality are crucial for long-term recovery. It is therefore important that the therapist discusses spirituality with the recovering addict. It is important to note that there is no hope without faith. People of old said that no person is an island unto himself. This is another way of saying that people need to support one another. Fellowship and human interaction are necessary ingredients in spirituality.

TRUE STORY: Joyce, a forty-four-year-old happily married mother of two and a professional accountant, lived a very busy life until injuries from an accident and subsequent surgeries turned her into an addict to pain medications. Several months into outpatient treatment, Joyce was advised to try yoga and meditation. Joyce tried yoga first, but because of her injuries, she opted to practice regular meditation instead. Joyce reported that meditation became a tonic for her spirit and helped her to relax. She further explained that meditation helped her to let go, particularly after a hectic day at the office. It should be noted that her therapist explained the differences between religion and spirituality to Joyce before she embarked on her journey.

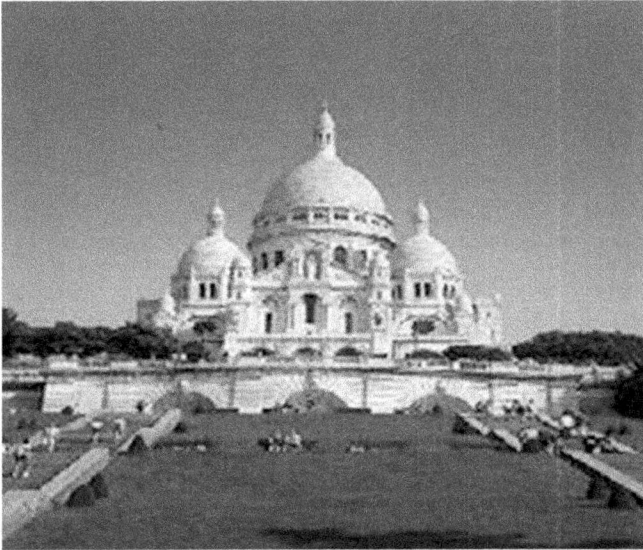

Religion and Spirituality : Sacred Heart Basilica - Paris

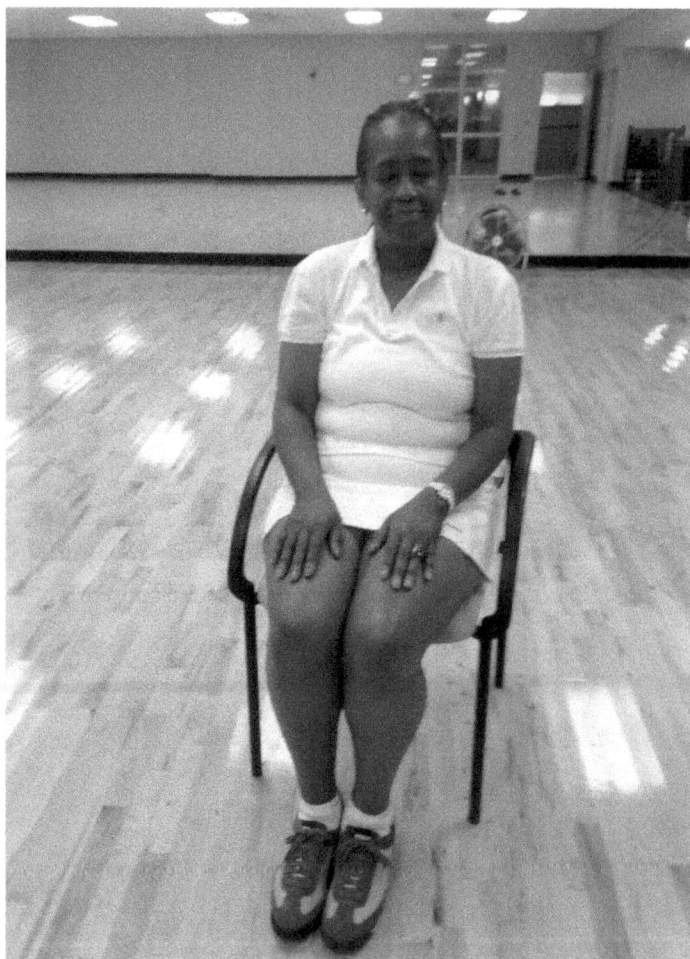

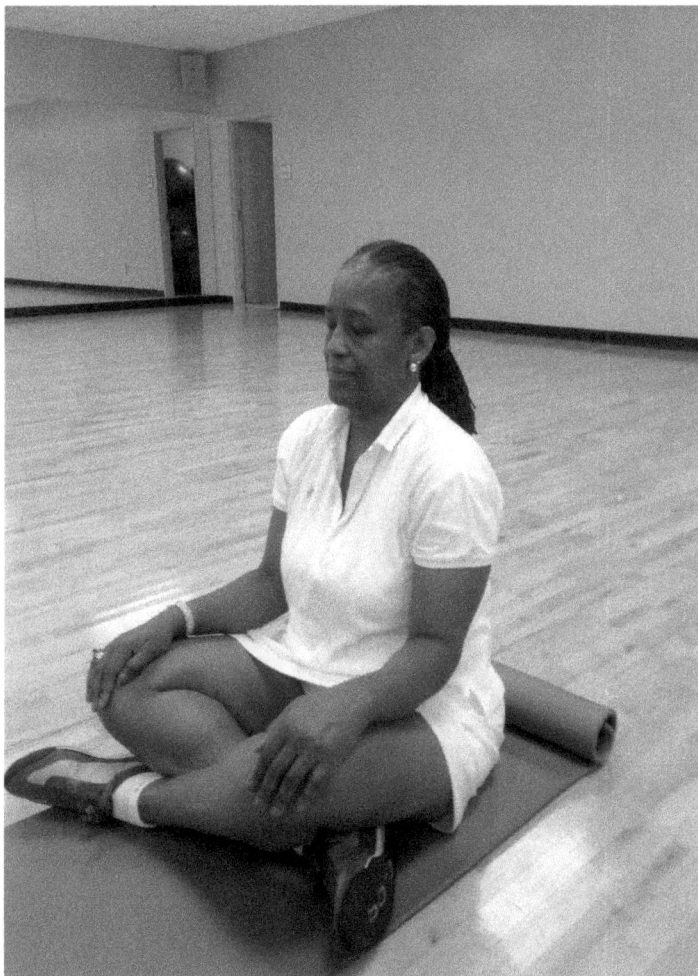

PICTURE OF MEDITATION POSES AND YOGA

Join a Sport Center for active lifestyle.

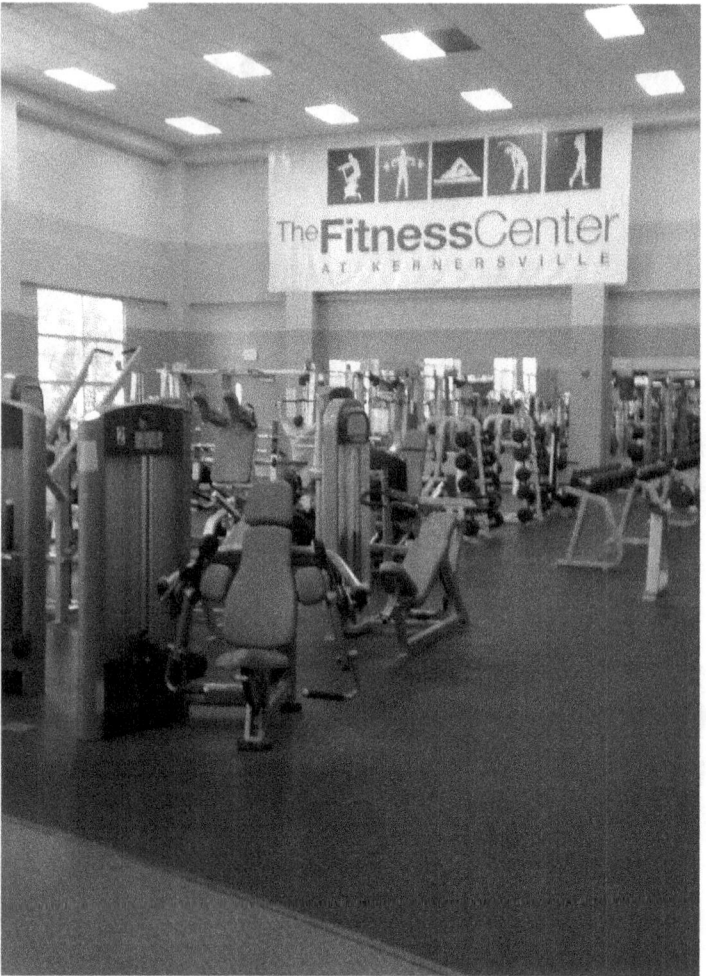

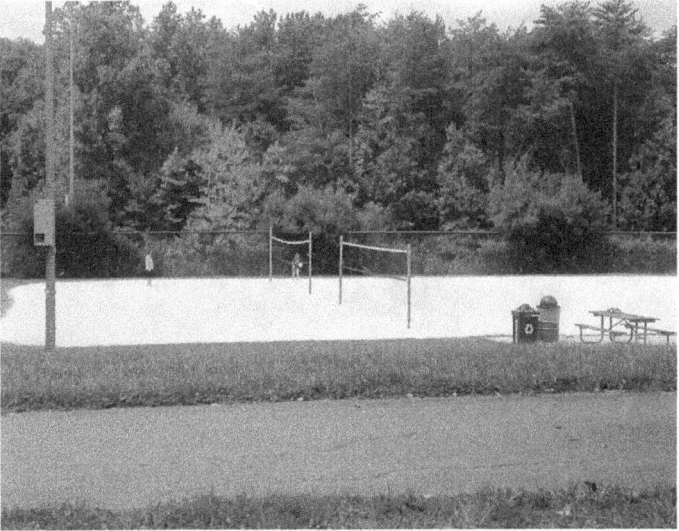

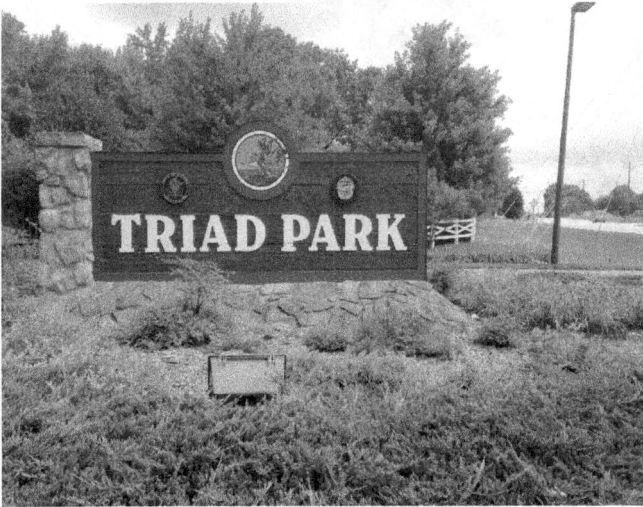

Public Park for walking and exercise.
Exercise, meditation, and yoga

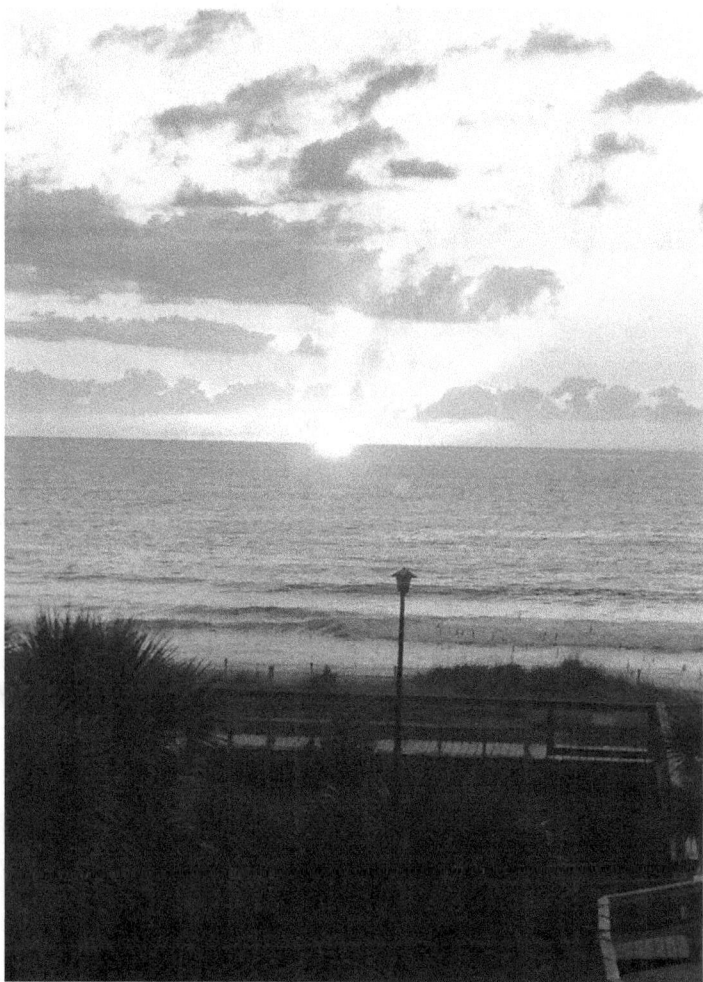

Practicing meditation facing the sunrise is very powerful.

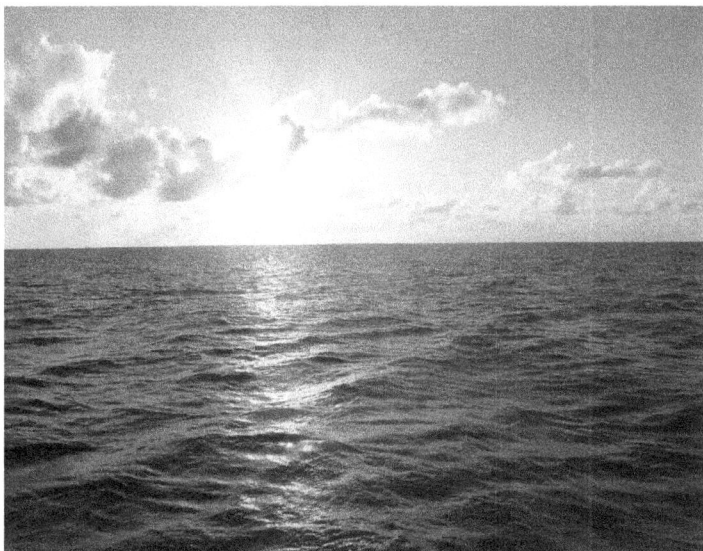

Practicing meditation facing a sunset is powerful!

EMOTIONAL LOGIC AND TRIGGERS

Past trauma is the key to understanding emotional logic and triggers. Under normal circumstances we expect small events to trigger small emotional reactions. It is the same for larger triggers. However, this is never so simple. When we experience a large emotional reaction to a small trigger, we are disturbed. The large emotional reaction is better understood when the past is considered. Triggers can be anything: something you see, hear, smell, taste, or touch.

Here are some steps to avoid triggers: watch body cues, avoid knee-jerk reactions, watch your feelings and write them down, look back into your past life, avoid transference (superimposed images of those who hurt you over the image of the person who triggered the reaction), address the original trauma, and choose to respond differently.

Note: *The therapist must understand the fact that past traumas are triggers for the recovering drug addict. The therapist should use psychodynamic therapy to help address the traumas of the past and then examine emotional logic and triggers with the recovering drug addict.*

TRUE STORY: Alfredo, a thirty-two-year-old white dancer and waiter, was abandoned as a baby. Alfredo spent years moving from one foster home to another until he turned eighteen. Alfredo suffered from separation anxiety for years, not knowing why or how to cope. One day Alfredo disclosed the details of his past life to his therapist. The therapist helped Alfredo to learn to cope with his anxiety symptoms and deal with the triggers.

TOPIC 14.

H-A-L-T (**H**UNGRY, **A**NGRY, **L**ONELY, **T**IRED)

The recovering addict must stay in touch with his or her feelings and needs. The onset of anxiety or a sudden drop in mood can be traced to our having forgotten to eat. Being hungry and tired can affect blood sugar levels, and this can cause anxiety and mood change.

It is best to take a little time out from our busy days to ask ourselves if we are feeling *Hungry*, *Angry*, *Lonely*, or *Tired*. There is a need to get in touch with our feelings in order to be healthy and abstinent. Once we know the cause—or causes—of what we are feeling, we can then make choices and take the appropriate action to address our needs for food, companionship, or rest.

Being hungry, angry, lonely, or tired leaves us more vulnerable to relapse. It is crucial that the recovering addict learns to pay attention to these inner signals and addresses issues in a manner that will enhance abstinence and serenity.

<u>Note:</u> *The therapist should train the recovering drug addict to recognize conditions such as hunger, anger, loneliness, and fatigue as possible triggers. The objective is to assist the recovering addict in recognizing physiological conditions that might send him or her back to using drugs.*

TRUE STORY: Drew, a twenty-nine-year-old white teacher, loved to socialize. Loneliness often led Drew into boredom and drug use. Drew was taught to prepare strategies on how to deal with boredom and loneliness. Thomas often got anxious and restless as soon as he felt hungry. Thomas learned to recognize this condition and to plan to eat at regular times.

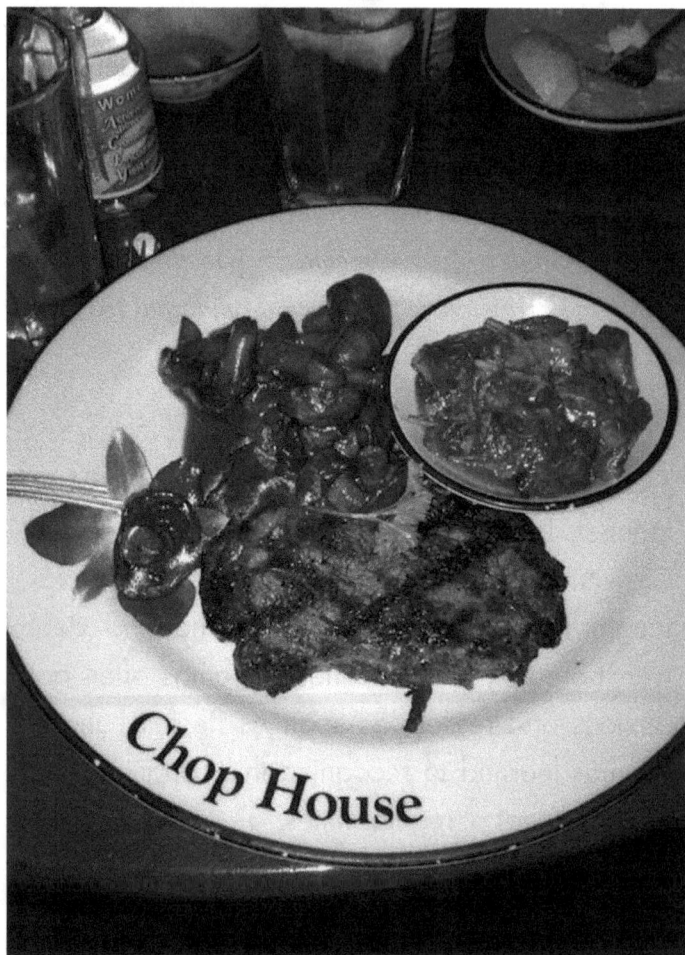

Eat quality food in small portions and at
regular hours for good health

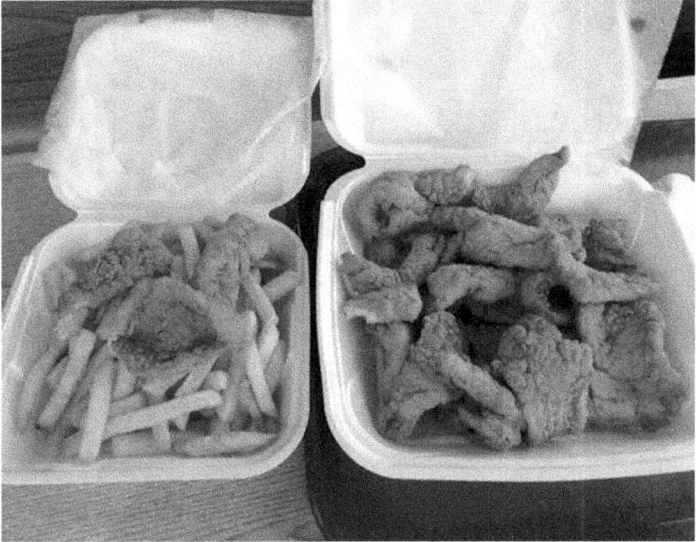

"You are whatever you eat." Cheap and tasty food may not be good for your health.

STRUCTURING ONE'S TIME

For the recovering drug addict, time management is crucial in coping with boredom. The goal is to focus on the activities that effectively give the greatest returns. Time management is important for recovering addicts in avoiding the snares of boredom and ultimately relapse.

Note: _The therapist should train the recovering drug addict to manage his or her time effectively._

TRUE STORY: A chronic drug addict often spends time chasing the drugs. Edward, a forty-two-year-old married father of two and a county government worker, was a chronic cocaine addict for many years. Once in treatment, Edward learned to structure his time doing something positive and constructive. Edward had to accept that boredom could lead him to use drugs. As a result, Edward starts each day by planning his activities for the whole day.

TOPIC 16.

HEALTHY ACTIVITIES

Healthy activities will equip the recovering addict with coping skills to help maintain abstinence. The recovering addict has to consider and adopt some or all of the following activities: relaxation, physical activity, and better nutrition. Healthy activities generate a physically and emotionally healthy life. Recreational activities help reduce stress and help the patient maintain a sense of balance in his or her life.

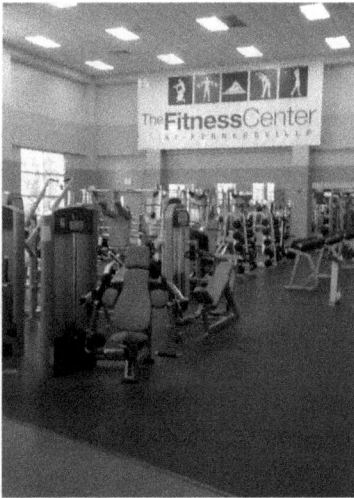

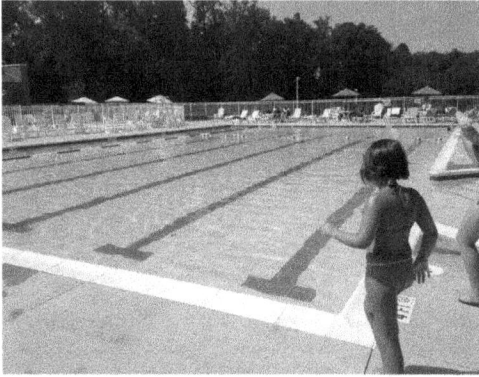

Daily exercise is good for your health

With help from the therapist, the recovering drug addict should explore the kinds of healthy recreational activities he or she used to enjoy prior to a life of addiction. The therapist, if possible, should encourage the patient to resume participation in such activities.

CAUTION: Although healthy activities can boost abstinence, the patient should check with his or her family doctor before engaging in any form of strenuous physical activity, except in cases where the patient is known to be healthy. Recovering addicts who indulge in physical activity cope better with boredom, thus avoiding triggers. Physical activities help lessen the severity of acute withdrawal symptoms.

How much healthy activity is enough? A moderate amount of physical activity is recommended. Studies show that moderate physical activity, performed daily, can substantially reduce the risk of heart disease, colon cancer, diabetes, and high blood pressure. Exercise also improves strength and endurance, controls weight, reduces stress and anxiety, and increases self-esteem.

Note: _The therapist must discuss the importance of healthy activities. The therapist should propose resources for healthy activities._

TRUE STORY: Pamela, a twenty-eight-year-old single pharmaceutical rep, suffered for many years from alcoholism. Pamela hid her addiction from her parents and lovers for years. Pamela was a workaholic. She lived for her job, and she never had time for anything else. Once in treatment, her therapist encouraged Pamela to engage in healthy activities to further help her recovery efforts. Pamela joined with a group of women who walked at a nearby public park. The women walked together, mostly on weekends. Pamela also joined a gym near her office.

TOPIC 17.

SHAME AND GUILT

Shame is defined as the tendency for someone to feel bad following a specific event. Shame is the emotion caused by the consciousness of guilt. People who have the tendency to feel shame when dealing with a variety of life problems are more likely to turn to alcohol and other drugs to cope with shame.

Guilt is the bad feeling that follows a specific behavior or action. Guilt is felt before shame.

Recovering drug addicts often leave behind wreckage or "burned bridges." It is crucial that the therapist helps the recovering drug addict learn to cope with persistent feelings of shame and guilt from his or her past.

Note: The therapist should discuss the effects of shame and guilt as triggers with the recovering drug addict and propose coping mechanisms.

TRUE STORY: Tim, a forty-five-year-old unemployed white male, was in treatment and making progress. However, Tim talked often about feeling guilt and shame for putting his parents through the agony of witnessing his chronic drug addiction and the wreckage of his life. The therapist validated Tim's feelings of guilt and shame but encouraged him to work harder for a successful treatment this time. A successful treatment would be a gift to his parents. The goal was for the therapist to work with Tim to prevent the feelings of shame and guilt from becoming an impediment to successful treatment.

THE COST OF ADDICTION AND PERSONAL INVENTORY

It is advisable that the recovering drug addict takes a personal inventory in order to recognize what he or she has been through and then plot a new path for the future. A thoroughly prepared inventory facilitates honesty with oneself and responsibility toward oneself and others, which in turn can foster greater self-acceptance. This exercise should be repeated during recovery. Studies show that each time the inventory is done, it becomes clearer—it shows increased honesty and improved self-awareness.

The recovering addict should look into the following: the effect of addiction on the patient, the effect of addiction on those around the patient, and the character defects in the patient that fed the addiction, such as insecurities, fears, anxieties, poor self-image, lack of confidence, excessive pride, controlling behavior, anger, and others.

Note: _The therapist might consider asking the recovering drug addict to prepare a list of the cost of his or her addiction. The recovering drug addict can then begin to realize the important losses of his or her life._

TRUE STORY: Ben, a forty-seven-year-old black man, was in treatment for a chronic cocaine addiction, and he was doing well. The therapist gave Ben an assignment: to put pen to paper and list the cost of his addiction. As Ben worked on the list, it got longer and clearer. Ben said that the cost of his addiction was shocking, considering the number of costly events and lost opportunities. Ben listed the loss of his inheritance, his house, his marriage, various jobs, and so on. Most importantly, Ben cried when he talked about the death of his trusted associate to a drug overdose, which happened while the two buddies were using drugs. Ben further stated that preparing a personal inventory helped him to fortify his determination to remain abstinent for a long time.

CHARACTER DEFECTS

The recovering drug addict should make a list of character defects, such as intolerance, minimizing, phoniness, self–centeredness, anger, resentment, covetousness, denial, false pride, procrastination, self–pity, impatience, intolerance, minimizing, and so on, and work hard to rid him or herself of such.

Note: *The therapist should give another assignment to the recovering drug addict: draw a list of his or her personal character defects.*

TRUE STORY: James, a thirty-eight-year-old self-employed black male, was an unrepentant procrastinator. James entered into treatment for his chronic use of marijuana. James had been abstinent for about six months when he started to work seriously on his character defects. James worked on being punctual and improving both his work and social ethics. James stated that it was difficult for him to adopt and adjust to socially acceptable characteristics. However, after mustering efforts to improve his character for some weeks, James started to receive compliments from people around him. James further explained that he is now used to receiving compliments rather than insults.

DEVELOPING A DRUG-FREE LIFESTYLE

Returning to a drug-free lifestyle can be a difficult project for a recovering addict. It is a given that the addict's past active drug-using life revolved around getting drugs, using drugs, and scoring drugs through association with fellow drug users. At the beginning of recovery, it is advisable for the recovering drug addict to establish a new social circle, a new residence (if possible), and healthy activities. It is important that the recovering addict cut off contact with all old associates. Volunteering and exploring spirituality are crucial activities for a recovering addict. Another part of developing a drug-free lifestyle is to establish a daily schedule or strict time-management regimen. Time management is needed to help the recovering addict manage his or her life for better health.

Note: _The therapist has to encourage the recovering drug addict to establish a daily schedule and adopt a drug-free lifestyle._

TRUE STORY: Tony, a twenty-nine-year-old white, unemployed veteran, served in the war in Iraq. After serving two tours of duty, Tony, who was silently suffering from PTSD, started drinking heavily and snorting cocaine. Tony had to seek treatment after an incident for which he was charged for assaulting his girlfriend. The girlfriend dropped the charges on the condition that Tony sought treatment. Prior to seeking treatment, Tony would go to bars to drink and hang out with his cocaine-snorting buddies. Once Tony got serious about treatment, he started going to church with his girlfriend and working out at the gym, and he stopped associating with his old friends.

TOPIC 21.

RETURNING TO SCHOOL OR WORK

Returning to active life is a good way to help a recovering addict regain control of his or her life. Whereas a return to work, or school, is a laudable outcome, it should happen deep into the recovery, once the patient is stable and capable. This is because a patient in the early stages of recovery is still quite vulnerable to stress, and the work or school environment could trigger relapse. The best time to return to work or school should be agreed upon between the patient and the therapist. Special attention must be paid to how the patient manages a stressful work or school environment. If a patient used cocaine to cope with stress at work, it is to be expected that he or she is likely to return to his or her old habit . If having ready cash was a major trigger for the patient, an early return to work and getting paid could cause him or her to relapse.

TRUE STORY: Brenda, a forty-two-year-old black single mother of two boys, entered into treatment for alcoholism. While in treatment, Brenda expressed the desire to return to school to work toward a degree in counseling in order to help other addicts. Brenda did not waste time in securing admission to a community college in her state. While working toward her degree, Brenda got a job as a peer support specialist, and soon she was sponsoring other recovering addicts.

TOPIC 22.

TRANSFERRING ADDICTIVE BEHAVIORS

Quite often, the addict trades one addictive behavior for another. People with addictive personalities have the tendency to transfer from one compulsive behavior to another. Whatever the behavior), the main concern is the compulsion to act, which becomes overpowering and destructive. This is because the behavior completely controls the addict's life, thus rendering it unmanageable. The patient must learn to recognize and take control of his or her life by shifting away from such behaviors. Using CBT (Cognitive Behavioral Therapy), the patient will learn to manage his or her life (behavior) so as to improve health. Even during recovery, the patient might compulsively attend several meetings daily. Whereas it is good to nurture this behavior in the early stages of recovery, the therapist must pay attention to help the patient abstain from compulsion.

Note: *The urge to switch from one addictive behavior to another is particularly great at the initial stage. The therapist should instruct and prepare the recovering drug addict to work hard at total abstinence and not substitute one addictive behavior for another.*

TRUE STORY: Following a random drug screen at a local methadone clinic, many patients tested positive for cocaine. These were patients who were receiving treatment for opioid dependence using methadone. The clinicians held a meeting to address this issue. What caught the clinicians by surprise was that those testing positive for cocaine did not use cocaine prior to entering treatment for opioid dependence. It was evident that their brains, having recovered from opioid dependence, were open to acquiring a new substance for pleasure.

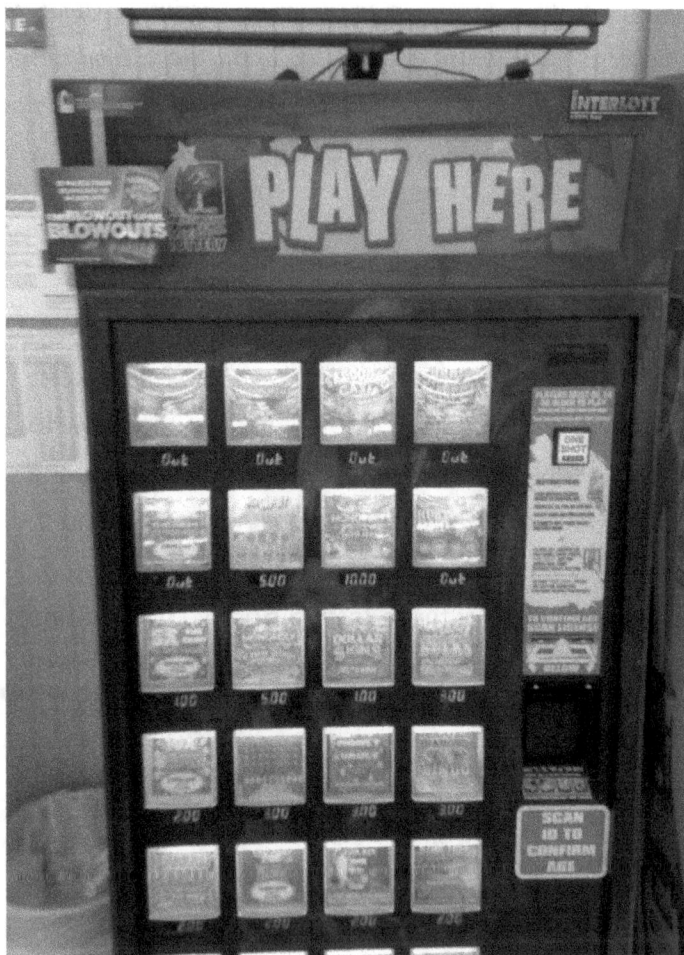

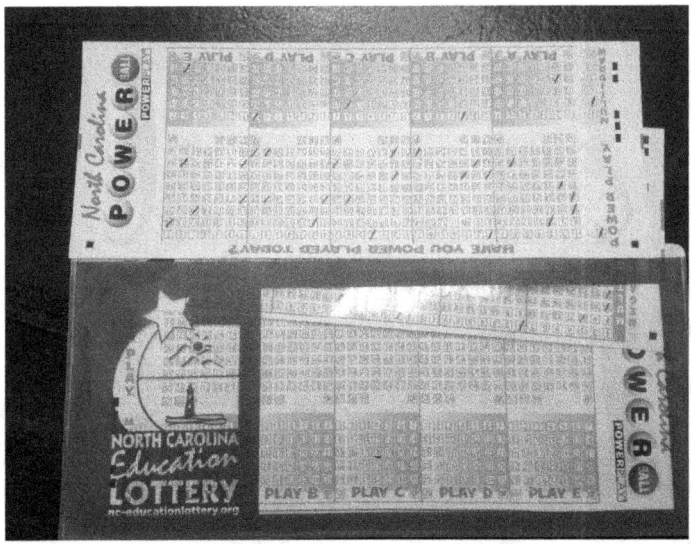

TOPIC 23.

RELAPSE PREVENTION

Relapse prevention is a necessary part of the aftercare treatment strategy. Relapse prevention was initially developed for the treatment of problem drinking, and it was adapted later for cocaine addicts. Using CBT, the patient learns to identify and correct compulsive behaviors. Relapse prevention is made up of a collection of strategies meant to train patients in self-control. The techniques are exploring the positive and negative consequences of maladaptive behavior, learning to recognize triggers and cravings at the early stage, learning to identify high-risk situations that could trigger relapse, and overall being proactive in order to avoid becoming trapped.

Research indicates that the skills individuals learn through relapse prevention therapy remain after the completion of treatment. In one study, most people who learned this cognitive-behavioral approach maintained the gains they made in treatment throughout the following year.

TRUE STORY: Debbie, a forty-five-year-old single white unemployed female, was a chronic heroin addict for fifteen years. She was abstinent for about ten years before she relapsed. The therapist working with Debbie soon identified her relapse triggers. It became evident that Debbie often relapsed whenever she was in contact with family members who did not approve of her lifestyle (Debbie was a lesbian). The strategy was to help Debbie avoid having frequent contact with her siblings until her relatives and siblings were able to accept her for who she was and not what they wanted her to be.

DRUG SCREENING

Therapists must endeavor to perform periodic urine sample testing to detect the presence of illegal substances. Drug testing is meant to encourage and monitor the drug addict in recovery. Drug screening should not be used as punishment for noncompliance with treatment program rules. Drug screening can be used as a tool to forestall relapse.

TRUE STORY: Random drug screening happens often in reputable clinics. Patients caught with illegal substances in their systems usually react negatively to the results. However, patients whose results came out as negative to the presence of illegal substances were elated to be classified as compliant.

MEDICAL CONSEQUENCES OF DRUG ABUSE

The chronic use or abuse of drugs cause severe health issues such as an abnormal heart rate, lung disease, constipation and stomach inflammation, bone disease, kidney failure, brain or neurological problems, disruption of hormonal production, cancer, premature birth or birth defects, other mental health problems, and death (sources: NIH, NIDA, and USFDA).

TRUE STORY: Chronic use of cocaine and/or marijuana can produce symptoms such as paranoia, depression, and hallucination. A patient became paranoid after binging on cocaine for several days. Jason was not known to suffer from paranoia until someone called 911 from the crack house. It was reported that Jason was talking about suicide and homicide. Jason was whisked to the ER, placed on a suicide watch, and kept for overnight observation.

MIXING ALCOHOL WITH MEDICATIONS

There are major health risks when alcohol is mixed with medications, for several reasons. Drowsiness can occur. Alcohol can potentially increase the effect of the medication, or produce other potentially harmful interactions. As well, keep in mind that some medications already contain up to 10 percent alcohol, alcohol can affect women differently than men, older people can be at greater risk, and alcohol and medications can interact harmfully, even when not taken at the same time.

TRUE STORY: A patient, Kathy, who herself was recovering from heroin addiction, discussed her concerns regarding her mother and her stepfather. Kathy stated that she had observed her mother and stepfather washing down their prescription medications with alcohol. The therapist explained to Kathy that mixing alcohol and drugs presents major health risks. The therapist further encouraged Kathy to tell her mother and step-father to seek help. Some days later, Kathy told her therapist that her mother and stepfather had told her that since the medications had been prescribed by their doctors and were not illegal drugs, they were fine. Some weeks later Kathy's mother passed out and had to be rushed to the hospital, where she later died. Not long after the death of Kathy's mother, Kathy's stepfather was also hospitalized and later died.

GLOSSARY OF MENTAL HEALTH / DRUG AND ALCOHOL ADDICTION CONDITIONS:

ADHD - Attention deficit hyperactivity disorder (ADHD) and attention deficit disorder (ADD) have symptoms that may begin in childhood and continue into adulthood. ADHD and ADD symptoms can cause problems at home, school, work, and in relationships.

ALCOHOL ABUSE - Alcohol abuse is defined as a pattern of drinking that results in one or more of the following situations within a twelve-month period:

- Inability to work, attend school, or take care of home responsibilities
- Drinking in situations that are physically dangerous (DUI or DWI)
- Involvement in alcohol-related legal problems (DUI or DWI)
- Relationship problems due to drinking

Heavy or chronic alcoholism can cause heart disease, liver disease, and even cancer. Treatment consists of medications and therapy in outpatient or residential settings.

ALCOHOL DEPENDENCE - When an alcoholic drinks compulsively, he or she is then dependent on repeated use of alcohol. Dependence has both physiological (tolerance and withdrawal symptoms) and psychological features. This disorder can be very disabling and distressing.

ANOREXIA NERVOSA (AN) - Anorexia nervosa is weight loss due to excessive dieting and exercise, sometimes to the point of starvation. Sufferers of AN are never satisfied with being thin enough. Considering themselves as "fat" can ultimately lead to extreme weight loss and death.

BIPOLAR DISORDER (highs and lows) – Sufferers of bipolar disorder (highs and lows) are prone to extreme mood swings between the two poles (polar: highs and lows). In the high phase, the sufferer has lots of energy, and he or she can be excessively functional. The sufferer has zero functionality in the low phase. Bipolar disorder is very serious and can cause risky behavior, such as suicidal thoughts or ideation.

BIOFEEDBACK - Biofeedback is used to harness the power of the mind and becoming more aware of what's going on inside the body to gain more control over health.

Researchers don't know exactly how or why biofeedback works. Biofeedback is known to promote relaxation, which can help relieve stress.

BINGE-EATING DISORDER - Binge eating disorder is characterized by regular episodes of extreme overeating and feelings of loss of control about eating that follow. Eating disorders typically develop during the teenage and young adult years. Eating disorders are much more common in girls and women. There is no known cause; however, eating disorders seem to coexist with psychological and medical issues such as low self-esteem, depression, anxiety, trouble coping with emotions, and substance abuse.

BULIMIA NERVOSA - Bulimia (say "boo-LEE-mee-uh") is a type of eating disorder. People with bulimia will eat a large amount of food in a short time (binge). Then they will do something to get rid of the food (purge). They might vomit, exercise too much, or use laxatives. Binge-eating gives sufferers a feeling of comfort. But binge-eating also creates bad feelings (such as guilt and shame), which cause them to purge.

CREATININE - Creatinine is a waste product that results from the normal breakdown of muscle tissue. As creatinine is produced, it's filtered through the kidneys and excreted in urine. Doctors measure the creatinine level in the blood as a test of kidney function. The kidneys' ability to handle creatinine is called the creatinine clearance rate, which helps to estimate the glomerular filtration rate (GFR), the rate of blood flow through the kidneys.

DEPRESSION - Depression is more than feeling sad. It is the intense feelings of sadness and other symptoms, like losing interest in things you enjoy. Depression is a medical condition and not a sign of weakness. It is treatable with medication and therapy.

DIZZINESS - Dizziness is a word that is often used to describe two different feelings. It is important to know exactly what you mean when you say "I feel dizzy," because it can help you and your doctor narrow down the list of possible problems.

> **Lightheadedness** is a feeling that you are about to faint or "pass out." Although you may feel dizzy, you do not feel as though you or your surroundings are moving. Lightheadedness often goes away

or improves when you lie down. If lightheaded-ness gets worse, it can lead to a feeling of almost fainting or a fainting spell (syncope). You may sometimes feel nauseated or vomit when you are lightheaded.

Vertigo is a feeling that you or your surroundings are moving when there is no actual movement. You may feel as though you are spinning, whirling, fall-ing, or tilting. When you have severe vertigo you may feel very nauseated or vomit. You may have trouble walking or standing, and you may lose your balance and fall.

DRUG ABUSE & DRUG ADDICTION - Use doesn't automatically lead to abuse, and there is no specific level at which drug use moves from casual to problematic. It varies by the individual. Drug abuse and addiction is less about the amount of the substance consumed or the fre-quency and more to do with the consequences of drug use. No matter how often or how little you're consuming, if your drug use is causing problems in your life—at work, school, home, or in your relationships—you likely have a drug abuse or addiction problem.

Common signs and symptoms of drug abuse
- Neglecting your responsibilities
- Using drugs under dangerous conditions or taking risks while high
- Getting into legal trouble
- Causing problems in your relationships

Common signs and symptoms of drug addiction
- Building up a drug tolerance
- Taking drugs to avoid or relieve withdrawal symptoms
- Loss of control over drug use
- Life revolves around drug use
- The abandonment of activities you used to enjoy
- Continued use in spite of wreckages

HIV/AIDS - Human immunodeficiency virus, or HIV, is the virus that causes AIDS. HIV/AIDS weakens a person's ability to fight infections and cancer. HIV transmission can occur with unprotected sex or with needle sharing (intravenous drug users). Symptoms of HIV vary widely. A person may have HIV symptoms or AIDS symptoms without knowing it until he or she gets HIV testing. There is no

HIV cure at this time, although medications can delay the onset of AIDS.

INSOMNIA - Insomnia is a sleep disorder that is character-ized by difficulty falling and/or staying asleep. People with insomnia have one or more of the following symptoms:

- Difficulty falling asleep
- Waking up often during the night and having trouble going back to sleep
- Waking up too early in the morning
- Feeling tired upon waking

There are two types of insomnia: primary insomnia and secondary insomnia.

- Primary insomnia: This means that a person is having sleep problems that are not directly associ-ated with any other health condition or problem.
- Secondary insomnia: This means that a person is having sleep problems due to medical condi-tions such as asthma, depression, arthritis, can-cer, heartburn, or pain.

MEMORY LOSS - Whether it is occasional forgetfulness or loss of short-term memory, there are many causes of memory loss. It is a problem that affects most people to a degree.

Common causes of memory loss include medications such as antidepressants, antihistamines, antianxiety medications, muscle relaxants, tranquilizers, sleeping pills, and pain medications. Excessive use of alcohol and drugs is a known cause of memory loss.

MIGRAINE/HEADACHES - Migraines and other types of headaches (be they tension headaches or sinus headaches) are painful and disruptive to normal life. Migraine symptoms include a pounding headache, nausea, vomiting, and light sensitivity. Headache remedies include various types of pain relievers. Migraine treatments may also include anti-nausea drugs and medications to prevent or stop headaches.

SLEEP-RELATED EATING DISORDER - This is characterized by abnormal eating patterns during the night. Although it is not as common as sleep walking, nocturnal sleep-related eating disorders can occur during sleepwalking. Sufferers can walk into the kitchen and prepare food without a recollection of having done so. If NS-RED occurs often enough, a person can experience weight gain and progress into an increased risk of type 2 diabetes.

OBESITY - Being obese is having too much body fat, which can adversely affect good health. Studies show that having too much body fat can lead to the development of type 2 diabetes, heart disease, high blood pressure, arthritis, sleep apnea, and stroke.

PANIC/ANXIETY DISORDER - Anxiety is a normal human emotion we all experience. But when panic and anxiety symptoms escalate into anxiety attacks and panic attacks, it may be an anxiety disorder. Anxiety disorders include generalized anxiety disorder, social anxiety, and panic disorder. There is excellent treatment available for anxiety attacks, as well as panic attack symptoms, including medication and psychotherapy.

SCHIZOPHRENIA - Schizophrenia symptoms include distorted thoughts and hallucinations (visual and auditory). Usually starting in young adulthood, schizophrenia can also cause the sufferer to feel frightened and paranoid.

To make a schizophrenia diagnosis, a psychiatrist evaluates symptoms, tests, and medical history, and prescribes medications and possibly psychotherapy (or other types of talk therapy) for proper schizophrenia treatment. New research is helping us understand this disorder better.

SAD - Seasonal affective disorder, or SAD, is a type of depression that affects a person during the same season each year. It commonly known that sufferers feel much better in the spring and summer.

STRESS MANAGEMENT - Stress is a silent killer. People who don't manage stress well can have headaches, stomach pain, sleeping problems, illness, and depression. Stress can be better managed by journaling, meditation, exercise, social activities, or engaging in a hobby. Heart attack survivors who anger easily or who are often stressed out may be setting themselves up for another, potentially fatal heart attack, a new study suggests.

==

Researched and prepared on 05/23/2007 and updated on 09/13/2010, on 01/19/2013 and on 02/11/2016 by:

Joseph Adegboyega (Dr. Joe), PhD, MAC, LCAS, CCS, SAP, Clinical Director, Jimekun & Associates LLC, Winston Salem, NC.

==

Bibliographic References:

Papers written by Dr. Mercer and Dr. Woody

Article by Peggy L. Ferguson, PhD

NIH publications

NIDA publications – Principles of Drug Addiction Treatment – A research-based Guide (3rd edition)

==

www.ingramcontent.com/pod-product-compliance
Lightning Source LLC
Chambersburg PA
CBHW060514280326
41933CB00014B/2957